I0425519

Personal Body Makeover

A Common-Sense Guide to
Weight Loss & Healthy Living

By: Bobby Whiteside

Personal Body Makeover

A Common-Sense Guide to Weight Loss & Healthy Living

Author: Bobby Whiteside

Copyright © 2019 by Bobby Whiteside

All rights reserved. This book or any portion thereof may not be reproduced or used in any manner whatsoever without the express written permission of the publisher except for the use of brief quotations in a book review.

Printed in the United States of America

First Printing, 2019

ISBN 9781097803507

Published by:

RJW Creations

Charlotte N.C. 28227

Contact: minthillbillymail@aol.com

To purchase copies through Amazon, go to:

www.personalbodymakeover.com

Credits:

Jacquelyn Whiteside – editor

Tina Lineberger – editing and photography

Follow me on YouTube

at: https://www.youtube.com/user/minthillbilly

Disclaimer

I am not a doctor, nutritionist, or a dietician. The information I provide in this book is based on my personal experience. Any recommendations I may make about weight training, nutrition, supplements or lifestyle is based on my own personal experience. All of the information provided should be discussed between you and your doctor because working out involves risks.

Before starting any new diet and exercise program please check with your doctor and clear any exercise and/or diet changes with them before beginning. I do not claim to help cure any condition or disease. I do not provide medical aid or nutrition advice for the purpose of health or disease nor do I claim to be doctor or dietitian.

Any product recommendation is not intended to diagnose, treat, cure, or prevent any disease. My statements and information have not necessarily been evaluated by the Food and Drug Administration.

I expressly disclaim responsibility to any person or entity for any liability, loss, or damage caused or alleged to be caused directly or indirectly as a result of the use, application or interpretation of any material provided to you as the reader of this book.

Dedication

To my parents Jack and Dianne Whiteside who brought me into this world. They raised me into the man I am today and have always been there for me even when I stumbled on the rocks of life. I love you.

Contents

"Every Champion Was Once a Contender Who Refused to Give Up." -Rocky Balboa

Preface

The Shortest Fitness Book Ever

This may turn out to be one of the shortest weight loss/fitness books ever written. I won't bore you with a lot of scientific content and pages upon pages of theories and analyses. I'm going to give it to you straight and to the point. There are plenty of books out there that dig deep into the subject of fitness and weight loss. I know because I have purchased several of these books and magazines over the years on this topic.

This is not rocket science and I want a book that you can pick up and read in its entirety in a few hours. I want you to be motivated to get started right away after closing the back cover upon completion of reading this book. I hope you will feel empowered to take control of your overall fitness and be willing to do whatever it takes to reach your personal goals.

My Vision for This Book

Earlier today, I responded to a comment on one of my YouTube videos that really touched me. The video was titled "My First 5K Run After Losing 50 lbs. in 3 Months"

The man left a comment congratulating me and also letting me know that my fitness videos have inspired him to start his own fitness journey. I was so pleased in knowing that my video had inspired someone to make a change in their life. For me, there is no better feeling than knowing that one of my videos has helped or motivated someone.

With that said, my vision for this book is to inspire as many folks out there as possible to make a positive change in their physical health and find the strength to maintain a healthy lifestyle. God Bless all that read this book and when you are finished please pass it on to others so it may help them as well.

Faith

I haven't always been the model Christian and I won't go into great detail of where I've fell short of His glory over the years in this fitness book, but I do believe that Jesus Christ is my Lord and savior. Having faith in Jesus has helped guide me through some rough times in my life and has also helped me with my personal fitness challenge. A relationship with Jesus will help guide you as well.

I've also found throughout this fitness journey that while walking it's also a good time to pray and talk to God. Here are a few verses from the Bible that I like to keep in mind:

Matthew 19:26 - But Jesus beheld them, and said unto them, with men this is impossible; but with God all things are possible.

Philippians 4:13 - I can do all things through Christ which strengthens me.

Introduction

About the Author

My name is Bobby Whiteside and I was born 51 years ago and raised in Charlotte NC. I am by no means an authority on fitness or weight loss but I can share with you my experiences and lessons learned over the years.

I grew up in a suburban neighborhood on the east side of Charlotte and it was a great experience with lots of fond memories. It was back in the day when kids played outside all day long with their friends. We played every sport imaginable and rode our bicycles everywhere we went. It was back before cell phones, cable TV, the internet, and the fear of some weirdo kidnapping a kid off the street in broad daylight. The only fear we had back then was being late for dinner. My childhood was truly a great time of my life and I still stay in touch via Facebook with all my old friends from the neighborhood.

I think I was around 12 years old when I got my first set of weights. It was the old plastic weights that were filled with concrete. My dad built me a weight bench out of wood, and we set up our own little home gym in the den of our split-level house.

Later in my teenage years we upgraded to some cast iron weights and a family friend gave us a heavy duty, homemade, steel weight bench and a bunch of muscle magazines from the 1960's. Those old magazines were a wealth of information for me as I journeyed though building a stronger body.

By the time I was in high school I had already had several years of weight training experience. I signed up for weight training in my sophomore year but ended up in P.E. class because the weight training class was reserved for athletes and was controlled by the coaches.

At some point during the year our PE class spent a week training on some old Nautilus equipment they had set up in a room on the second level of the gymnasium. I naturally excelled at using that old equipment and loved every minute of it. At the end of the week, Coach Matthews pulled me aside and asked if I had any plans of playing football next year. I told him yes and that I would have played this year but I worked with my dad over the summer building houses so I could buy a car. He said, Let's get you transferred into weight training. He told me to go talk with the head football coach, Alan Sitterle, down in the 400 building.

Later that day, I went to Coach Sitterle's classroom and told him that Coach Matthews had sent me. After our discussion he allowed me to change my schedule and begin weight training the following week. The last thing he said to me was " We will put some muscles on you, so you won't have to wear those padded jackets around school."

It didn't take me long to excel in weight training. By the end of my 10th grade year my total max out of Bench press, Squat, deadlift, and power clean was over 1300 lbs.

The following year, I did play football and was still enrolled in weight training class. I made my biggest gains during this my junior year. By the end of the year I had excelled into the 1600lb club and received the most prestigious award in my mind which was a 1600 lb. t-shirt reserved only for football players. I was only the second person ever to receive a 1600 lb. shirt in that school's history, and I also set the all-time school power clean record that year at 325lbs.

At the sports awards banquet later that year I received a trophy for the most improved weightlifter that year. I still have that trophy and what's left of that 1600 lb. t-shirt that I wore with pride for years.

Since those days of being in excellent shape I haven't always stayed on the straight and narrow of my physical health. Life sometimes takes control and we find little time to do the things we need to stay in top shape. Over the years I've been on several health kicks to get back into shape and had good success for a while. I even did the EAS challenge when I was about 30 years old and got down to 6.2 percent bodyfat. Getting focused and disciplined to achieve a goal has never been a problem for me but, maintaining that consistency has been. I think a lot of us struggle with staying on the wagon when it comes to our health.

After 51 years I think I have finally got the right mindset and the right program to make this the final lifestyle change for me. In this book I will try to instill in the reader these principles so that you too can get to your healthy weight and maintain a healthy lifestyle.

Chapter One
Mindset

Goal Setting

Setting a goal to lose weight sounds easy, right? Thousands of people every year on New Year's make a resolution or a goal to lose weight in the new year. Most fail and here is why. Just saying, "I'm going to lose weight" is not a goal. That statement is a vague thought.

When setting a goal, whether it be to lose weight or save money or any other objective, there has to be a plan. The more detailed the plan is the more probable it is you will reach the goal you set.

Let's say you were setting a goal to save money. You need to define this objective in greater detail. Here is a series of questions that need to be answered to start putting together the plan.

- How much money do you want to save? (define the amount)
- When will this money be in my possession? (set a date)
- What expenses can you cut out of your budget? (i.e., cable TV, Starbucks, dining out, etc.)
- What items around the house can I sell? (i.e., boat, collectables, toys, clothes, etc.)
- Can I get a second job, part-time for a few months?

When you start answering these questions you will be on your way to making this goal possible.

Enough about money. I was using that as an example, but let's get on the subject of fitness goals. Along with a well thought out, detailed plan there will always be give and take with any goal. This is a must in any fitness goal whether it's to lose weight, build muscle, add strength, or run faster. There will be things that you will have to give up or at least learn to control. I'm mainly speaking of certain food or drinks that will have to be regulated if you want to see results. I will get into this subject further and with more clarity in another chapter.

Over the years, I've had many different kinds of fitness goals from my strength training goals back in high school to my most recent weight loss challenge. Each type of goal requires a different game plan, but since most people purchasing this book are probably desiring to lose weight and get healthy, I will focus on the latter.

Let's go back to Christmas of last year (2018). The kids were home for Christmas, and I was cooking great meals every day. We had bacon and waffles several mornings. One night I deep fried some chicken legs for dinner and the list goes on. We were eating good, or should I say not so good in a healthy sense.

Now I'm not saying that I got fat over Christmas break because of my cooking, but I did step on a set of scales and to my surprise I weighed over 285lbs. 286.6 to be exact and that was the heaviest I have ever been in my life. I didn't feel healthy and didn't like the site of my naked self in the mirror when I stepped out of the shower. I was also losing flexibility. It was getting more difficult to bend over to tie my shoes. I knew then that it was time to do something about my weight before it started causing some major health problems.

After that reality check, I set my only goal for 2019. My goal was to lose down to 230 lbs. It had been many years since I weighed 230 lbs., but I remember that was a good weight for me. Here is the following plan that I put together before January 1, 2019:

- Goal: I want to lose weight down to 230 lbs. in 2019 (no specific date to reach)

- Diet: I will cut out soft drinks, sweet tea and replace those with drinking water (8 oz. soft drink allowed in the morning).
- Exercise: I will walk daily and track my progress on the "Map my Walk" phone app.
- I will tell everyone what I'm doing so I will be held accountable. (I announced it to 17,000, subscribers on my YouTube channel as well.)
- I will step on the scales daily and micromanage my progress and track weekly results.
- I will announce my results to my YouTube family monthly.
- I will do some light weightlifting and heavy bag workouts 2 times per week.
- I will exercise proper portion control of my food and minimize white foods (i.e., sugar, salt, pasta, potatoes).
- I won't eliminate anything from my diet that I like but will control the portion size and frequency.
- I will be disciplined in sticking to the above guidelines to reach my goal.

Folks, this is what the outline of my Goal looked like on January 1st of this year. Notice that there is a clear weight that I wanted to reach sometime in 2019. This type of plan works! It may not work as fast for some people, but it will work.

Getting Tough

August 1st, 1985, it was the first official day of football practice at the High School that I attended. Before the first of two practices started that day, our coach, Rusty Jester, gathered all the prospective players for a meeting on some wooden bleachers near the practice field.

Coach Jester put his clipboard down, stood and faced all of us young men and proceeded with a sermon that every teenage boy should hear. I don't recall everything he said that day, but I do remember the following as if it were yesterday.

Coach said, "This is one of the biggest groups I've had on opening day of practice in all my years of coaching. There are over 120 of you out here today and I'll bet there are more boys that go to this school that wish they were out here trying out with you."

He went on to say, "I know from experience that after the next two weeks of two-a-day practices I will lose 30 to 40 of you. You will quit this team. You will quit because it's too hard or too tough." He went on to say, "120 players are more than I need to make our JV and Varsity teams. Most coaches have to cut players, but I'm not cutting anyone. If you make it through the next two weeks you are on the team."

Coach Jester looked us over harshly and said, "Don't Quit! If you quit this team you will quit things in life like a job or a marriage every time things get too tough for you to handle."

After the sermon was over, he blew his whistle and we all proceeded to the practice field. The first drill that day was 40-yard wind sprints. We were divided in groups of four or five. He blew that whistle to start us about 10 yards apart from one another. By the time you got to the other end there was little time to catch your breath before you were headed back the other way. This went on for what seemed like an hour before we moved on to a different drill.

After a few weeks the two-a-days were over and there were some that fell by the wayside, but I remained. I endured what seemed like torture both my junior and senior years. Both years I played through the pain of shin splints till they finally got better in mid-August.

As difficult as two-a-days were in the hot, August, Carolina sun, I wouldn't trade the lessons I learned those summers for anything. Coach Rusty Jester had a lot of influence on my mental and physical toughness.

Excuses? You Have None

It must have been about mid-January when I had stopped by the local park for my morning walk. I remember looking at the weather app on my phone and seeing that it was 23 degrees outside. I came close to not getting out of my truck, but I decided to at least walk one lap around the asphalt track.

As I began walking, I spotted a little old lady walking on the track. I had seen her out here before. However, on this morning, it was 23 degrees and she was the only other person out walking. I soon caught up with her and decided to speak to her. I said, "Good morning", and she replied back. "I said do you mind me asking how old you are?" She replied, "I'm 80 years old." I smiled and said, "God Bless you for being out here walking on this cold morning." She told me that she has been walking for years. I proceeded in telling her that I just started walking to lose weight. Her reply, "Walking is the best thing for you."

We said our good-byes and I continued walking that morning with a new pep in my step. Having that short conversation with her really motivated me. I ended up walking over two miles that morning. What started out to be just one lap around the track ended up being my longest walk so far at that point in my journey.

I kept thinking to myself, if an 80-year-old lady can get out and walk on a 23-degree day, then I have no excuse. From then on, every time the weather was cold or even a light rain, I would think about that 80-year-old lady.

Yes, I even walked in the rain on several days in February. I put on my cowboy hat and raincoat and got out there and Made it Happen. You Have No Excuse!

Negative Influences

I have discovered in life that no matter what you do or accomplish there will always be those who try to bring you down. Most of the time this negativity comes from our family and closest of friends. It makes perfect sense that it would be friends and family because our enemies never come around as the old saying goes. There will be those that will say you can never reach your fitness goal for one reason or another. Then they will elaborate on how a particular diet or program didn't work for them and that you should go ahead and give up and not waste your time. They will also remind you of someone they knew or heard of that was in great physical shape and died from a heart attack or some other medical condition. Negativity can be overwhelming at times and it's a stab to your heart when the ones closest to you are the ones trying to bring you down.

There is only one way to deal with the forces of negativity and that is to block it out. Listen to what the Doubting Thomas's and Negative Nancy's are trying to tell you with a smile on your face. Then you go out and use that as the fuel to power your mission. Let those harsh words build the armor that will make you bulletproof and unstoppable.

In the 1980's I was watching an interview with Junior Johnson on television. At the time, he was the top car owner of the Nascar Winston Cup division. I believe he was the first car owner to field two cars in every race. Junior Johnson came from humble beginnings in North Wilkesboro, North Carolina. In his younger years he ran moonshine and eventually began racing stock cars. Although he was a well-respected driver in the 1960's his ultimate success was in being a car owner. He was at the top of his career as he sat there being interviewed for this television program. When asked the question of how he became so successful and innovative as a car owner, Junior Johnson said something to the effect that "every time he was told he couldn't do something, or it couldn't be done, he would darn sure prove them wrong."

It's that Junior Johnson type of tenacity that you will need to overcome any negativity that comes your way. Don't push these people out of your life if they have a negative comment or two because at the end of the day, they are still your loved ones. Remember it's just human nature and some don't realize that words can hurt. Learn to take the negative and fuel the positive that will drive you to reach your goals.

"Take Pride in How Far You Have Come. Have Faith in How Far You Can Go" - Unknown

Chapter Two
Getting Started

Making time for you

I've heard a lot of people over the years say, "I don't have time to work out". Another statement they say is, "At the end of my day I'm too tired to work out".

Folks, these are the kind of excuses that will lead to failure. I bet these people could find some time to work out if they would get their butt out of bed in the morning instead of snoozing the alarm clock seven times. Maybe they could find time in the evening if they didn't have to watch every reality series television has to offer each night of the week.

Making time for yourself is just as important as setting the goal to lose weight. You will have to spend some time strategizing a point in the day where you can exercise. This needs to be a time slot that is open every day for you. You may not workout, walk or run every day, but have this time open just for you. If it is a rest day then spend that time reading some fitness articles online or watching some of the amazing weight loss stories of others on YouTube.

Personally, I love to walk every morning and sometimes I incorporate some running with my walk or ride my bicycle afterwards. Working out in the morning gives me a feeling of accomplishment that carries on through the day. If my day is getting busy, I don't have to wonder if I'm going to have time to work out later because I've already done it.

I've read many books over the years about successful people and one characteristic that they all seem to have is they get up very early in the morning. Most have a planned routine and they stick to it daily. They are in control of their day instead of the day controlling them. Find your timeslot and declare it your personal time.

Equipment you will need

The topic of equipment needed to exercise and get in shape can be overwhelming. Just flip through the TV channels any given day and you will find infomercials advertising the latest and greatest piece of equipment or program that you need to purchase now in order to get the tv discount. It's enough to make your brain turn to mush.

The truth is that you can get excellent results with no specialized equipment at all. You don't need any equipment to walk around the block of your neighborhood or to do push-ups, free squats, or lunges in your living room. For that matter you could double bag a couple of can goods from your cabinet and perform some curls, shoulder raises, and triceps kickbacks while standing in your kitchen. Don't get caught up in thinking you need some magical piece of equipment or program to achieve your goals.

If you plan on purchasing some equipment, then use resources such as Craigslist or the Facebook marketplace to find some great deals on used equipment. The folks that have fell off the fitness wagon are eager to get rid of the unused treadmill or stationary bike in their living room that has become a coat rack. You can also find great deals on free weights, including dumbbells and benches. Even if the weights are ugly and have a little rust on them, you can always clean them up and spray a coat of paint on them to make them look new again. When it comes to electrical equipment, such as treadmills and so forth, pay careful attention to the condition and operation before purchasing. One thing to check out closely on a treadmill is the belt. Find the point on the belt where it is seamed together and check for fraying on the underside. That will give you a good idea of how much it has been used.

There is another alternative and that is joining a Gym. I personally don't like Gyms because with it comes the "Gym-Life" as I like to call it. Most people spend more money on the clothing they wear to the gym than I spend on my whole wardrobe. It's insane the way most gyms have become a meat market or place to meet your next girl or boyfriend. I don't need all that craziness in my life and besides the time you spend driving back and forth to the gym can be the time spent working out.

Chapter Three
Diet & Exercise

Diet, Nutrition, and Supplements

As I mentioned previously, I am by no means a nutritionist, nor do I have any formal education in this area. There is plenty of information about this topic in print and online. Do all the research you can and consult a doctor or specialist for any advice for your situation.

What I can offer you is years of my personal experience and a common-sense approach to diet, nutrition, and supplements.

Let's start with supplements. The only supplement that I currently take is a multivitamin for men over 50. The only other thing that could be categorized as a supplement is the Whey Protein Powder that I use to make protein shakes. I use the Elevation brand protein powder that is sold at Aldi. I found it to be the least expensive and it tastes great for a mid-morning meal or an evening snack. Instead of reaching for a bag of chips or a bowl of ice cream I find that a shake curbs my hunger till the next meal.

In the past I have used a variety of sports supplements, including specialty vitamins, liver tablets, creatine, rip fuel and some I've probably forgotten about. I've never taken any legal or illegal steroids in my life and I strongly recommend you don't either. Some of these supplements advertise that no problems can occur and then we all find out later down the road that the effects can cause long term health problems. These products can be very effective but also very expensive. Unless you are prepared to continue spending the big money on these items you may see a decline in your results.

When most people hear the word diet, they think of eating less food and going hungry. I want you to think of the word diet as a purposely changed menu to help fuel your body properly to get maximum performance. I don't want anyone to compare dieting to hunger. If you are hungry then it's time to eat something. If you ignore your body telling you this, your brain will put your metabolism on lockdown. This is like your brain saying, "Hey, we are not getting any food so don't release the fat cells for energy. We need to ride this out until we get some food."

Now let's talk about changing the menu and by this, I mean start eating healthier foods and stop eating all the crap foods or at least minimize their consumption. I don't want anyone to totally give up anything that they really like to eat or drink. By doing this you are setting yourself up for failure because one day you're going to eat that bag of chips and feel like you failed yourself. This could turn into a whole big tailspin that makes you give up and say I'll never be able to reach my goal.

Maybe it's easier for me to tell you what I did to change my menu or diet for losing weight. I used to drink a lot of soft drinks and sweet tea. I probably took in well over 1000 calories a day in my liquid intake. I traded in the soft drinks and tea for water. I still allow myself eight to ten ounces of good ole Mountain Dew first thing in the morning. The next biggest thing I cut out was chips, crackers, cookies, and other easy to consume snack foods from a bag or box. I still allow myself these items, but they are no longer the go-to item in-between meals or late at night. If I need a little something to tie me over, I'll have a protein shake or a piece of fruit. To make these kinds of snacks easier to access quickly, I already have a watermelon or cantaloupe cut up in a bowl, in the refrigerator. Instead of making a big mess with a blender or magic bullet I mix my protein shakes in a solo cup with a butter knife. After I drink the shake, I toss the cup in the trash. Done, no clean up required.

I've heard it said before that all the healthy food is on the outside wall around a grocery store and all the crap food with preservatives is up and down all the aisles. The more I thought about that I realized that it's a true statement. On the outside walls of a store are the fresh fruits and vegetables, meats and fish, and all your dairy products such as milk, eggs and butter. There are still some good things on the middle isles such as dried beans, rice, oats, and grains. Although, I have cut back on what I like to call the white foods (sugar, salt, pasta and potatoes), I did decide to start baking my own bread. I found a couple of easy recipes and after a few attempts my bread now turns out perfect every time. Homemade bread has no preservatives so that's a plus for those of us looking for a healthier option.

Portion control and spacing your meals apart are two of the most important aspects to successfully losing weight. You will need to control your portion size at every meal. No more eating a whole large pizza in one sitting and then feeling miserable for the next three hours. One thing I started doing was only filling my dinner plate to the inner ring of the plate instead of having food falling off the edges as I carried it to the table. Go ahead and eat a conservative portion at every meal and then walk away, even if that means you are still feeling a little hungry. Wait 30 minutes and if you're still hungry then eat a little more. It takes a while for your stomach to communicate to your brain that "I've had enough down here! Stop putting food in the mouth." If you can get use to eating this way you will not miss those times when you overate and felt miserable afterwards.

Along with portion control it's better to split your meals into several smaller meals throughout the day. Five or six smaller meals instead of two or three larger ones can help boost your metabolism and keep the fat burning process rolling along.

Like I said before, I'm not a nutritionist but when I think of nutrition, I think of the four food groups that we were taught in school. If you don't remember, they are the milk and dairy group, the meat group, the fruit and veggie group, and the bread and cereal group. I recommend that you design your diet using foods from all four groups. I think God intended it that way for us to sustain a healthy diet.

Water - Drink Plenty of it!

The topic of drinking water is important enough that I made a separate sub heading on the subject. Drinking plenty of water in place of soft drinks and sweet tea has been a major part of my success. I have always had a weakness for these sugar-filled drinks and up until my fitness challenge I was probably consuming over 1000 calories a day from these drinks. As part of the outline for my fitness challenge I decided to trade in the soft drinks and sweet tea for water. This has proven to be a tremendous part of achieving some awesome weight loss results. In the first week of my challenge back in January, I immediately started noticing some changes in my body. Along with losing over 14 lbs. in the first week, I felt better in general. My stomach didn't have that bloated feeling all the time and I noticed that I had more energy and less body aches.

I did a little research on the internet and found a few of the positive things about drinking water that the experts say. Along with promoting healthy weight management and weight loss the experts say it flushes out toxins from the body. Increasing brain power and boosting energy are a few more attributes of drinking water. Water can also aid in preventing headaches, cramps, and improve your skins complexion.

Drinking plenty of water is an absolute necessity to initiate into your fitness plan. I personally drink over a gallon per day and sometimes more during the summer months. One thing we started doing at my household is filtering the tap water into a pitcher that stays in the refrigerator. I can't stress enough the importance of drinking more water and cutting down on soft drinks. I don't believe I would have made near the progress I have if I hadn't made the switch.

Cardio- Walking, Running, Cycling, and Weight training

I define Cardio as any type of exercise that brings your heart rate up. This exercises your heart which helps to prevent a number of health issues and generates fat loss. The research that I've found says 20 to 30 minutes of low intensity exercise daily can aid in heart health. This amount of time spent exercising daily can also produce some amazing fat loss results as well.

Another thing I've found through my experience is that it's better to do cardio in the morning after fasting all night than in the evening after you have taken in the majority of your calories for the day. I read in a journal one time that 20 minutes of cardio in the morning yields the same fat loss results as 60 minutes in the evening. When exercising in the morning on a near empty stomach, your body can break into releasing the fat storage cells sooner. I have used this method and it seems to work better for me.

There are many different ways to get a good cardio workout. Swimming, walking and cycling are a few of lowest impact exercises on your body. This is important to keep in mind for us older folks that have some discomfort in our joints, etc. Running, cross fit, jumping rope, and high rep weight training are some other exercises that can produce good results as well.

My personal favorite cardio exercise is walking. During my weight loss journey, I walked over 200 miles in three and a half months in reaching my goal weight of 230 lbs. I lost an amazing 56.6 lbs. along the way. Although I worked out with weights and did some heavy bag training early on in my journey, it was the daily walks that I stuck to religiously. After the first month or so I had worked my way up to walking five miles at a time on some days. I even got the courage to sign up for a 5k run that you will read about in another chapter.

I want to touch on the topic of weight training as a cardio workout. Most people think of weight training as a way to build muscle, but it can also be just as effective or more so in burning fat. In weight training most folks target certain muscle groups in a single workout. An example of this would be one day they will work on upper body and the next day they would work on lower body. There are even more variations to that routine as well. Some will split the upper body into two groups and that would add an additional day in your routine.

I have found for a good weight/cardio workout to work as many groups in one day with light weights, high repetitions, and shorter rest time in between sets. This can generate an awesome cardio workout. You can also apply super sets in your training. By this, I mean going from one exercise to another without any rest. I recommend choosing two movements that target different muscle groups. An example of this would be performing a set of bench press and then immediately beginning a set of half squats. After the set of half squats rest for a minute or so and repeat.

When using weight training as a way to cardio, you are not focusing on burning out a muscle group. Your main focus is getting your heart rate up and sustaining it throughout your workout. Along with getting a great cardio workout you are also toning and strengthening muscles. Another benefit to weight training is that after the workout is over, your body will continue burning calories longer thereafter than walking or other low impact exercises.

No matter what type of cardio you choose to put in your program the most important thing is that you do something. Get your body moving daily!

"Sometimes if you want to see a change for the better, you have to take things into your own hands." -Clint Eastwood

Chapter Four
Workout Examples

Examples of Work Out Routines

In this chapter I will give some examples of different exercises and routines you may want to initiate into your training. These examples will cover walking, running, cycling, heavy bag training, and weight training.

Walking

You folks already know how much I love to walk, and I feel it is a very effective, low impact exercise for almost everyone who is trying to lose weight. One thing I don't believe I've mentioned enough is the app on my phone that I use to track my walking. I use the Under Armor sponsored app called "Map My Walk". This app will track your distance via GPS and keep a timer running. The app also gives you an average speed per mile, as well as an estimate of calories burned. I'm sure there are other apps out there that provide this same information, but I started using "Map My Walk" and I really like it. You can also switch the screen over to a running or mountain biking setting as well. The app will also store long term data so you can go back and look at how much you walked, ran, or cycled in a given time frame. I definitely recommend downloading this app on your phone.

Walking Routine

Week 1 - Walk a mile each day or whatever you feel comfortable with this first week. After the first day determine from the app your average pace per mile. Try to increase your pace a little each day during the first week.

Week 2 - Walk 1.5 miles each day this week.

Week 3 - Walk 1.75 miles each day this week and try to increase your pace each day.

Week 4 - Walk 2 miles each day.

This is just an example. You can see the direction I'm proposing. You may only be able to start off at a half of a mile in the beginning. You will decide what works for you and declare your starting point. One thing to keep in mind is walking at least 20 to 30 minutes a day will get the fat burning process rolling along.

Running Routine

Up until recently it had been a long time since I picked my heels up and ran anywhere. I had to start off running short distances and walking in-between. This is the only way I can explain how to start running. You have to cycle between running and walking with the emphasize on increasing the running time until you build yourself up to running. You just have to work at it at least three times per week. I usually incorporate my runs on Mondays, Wednesdays, and Fridays.

Cycling

I really enjoy riding my bicycle and I try to ride it a few times per week after a long walk. If you choose to use cycling as your only means of exercise you would go about it in the same fashion as walking. I would ride daily and slowly increase my distance daily. When I was a kid, I rode a bicycle everywhere I went. I bet I averaged ten miles per day.

Weight Training

I'm going to provide some sample workouts below assuming that you have a basic weight set. I would recommend a barbell set with a few hundred pounds, a variety of dumbbells, and a bench that has the ability to incline. It's also a good idea to have someone that can act as a spotter on certain exercises.

Basic Weight Workout for Beginners

In this workout we will target all muscle groups in a single workout. This workout will be performed twice a week. Monday and Thursday would be an example of splitting up the training days. Each of the movements I list below will be further explained on how to perform them later in this chapter.

Bench Press - 3 sets of 10 repetitions

Half Squats - 3 sets of 10 repetitions

Standing Barbell Curl - 3 sets of 10 repetitions

Military Press - 3 sets of 10 repetitions

Bent over Barbell Row - 3 sets of 10 repetitions

Dumbbell Triceps Press - 3 sets of 10 repetitions

With these 6 exercises you will touch nearly every muscle in your body. Be careful not to overdo it on your first work out. You should feel some soreness in the days following but I don't want you to be in severe pain. Years ago, I had started back into a program and definitely over did it. My legs were so sore and tender I could barely walk the next day.

Intermediate Workout

This routine will require you to work out four times per week. The work outs will be split into an Upper body and a Lower body work out. You will perform the upper body workout on Mondays and Thursdays. The Lower body workout will be performed on Tuesdays and Fridays.

Upper Body Workout (Mondays and Thursdays):

Bench Press - 3 sets of 10 repetitions

Barbell Curls - 3 sets of 10 repetitions

Bent Over Barbell Row - 3 sets of 10 repetitions

Military Press - 3 sets of 10 repetitions

Dumbbell Triceps Press - 3 sets of 10 repetitions

Dumbbell Flies - 3 sets of 10 repetitions

Lower Body Workout (Tuesdays and Fridays):

Half Squats - 3 sets of 10 repetitions

Calf Raises - 3 sets of 10 repetitions

Crunches - 3 sets of 10 repetitions

Lunges - 3 sets of 10 repetitions

Leg Lifts - 3 sets of 10 repetitions

Leg Curls - 3 sets of 10 repetitions

Advanced Workout

This workout program will be a six-day split routine. There will be a workout for the Back and Biceps. There will be a workout for Legs and Abs and a workout for Chest, Shoulders, and Triceps. Each one of these routines will be performed twice a week. Thus you will only have one rest day per week. The Chest, Shoulder, and Triceps workout will be performed on Mondays and Thursdays. The Back and Bicep workout will be on Tuesdays and Fridays. The Leg and Abs workout will be performed on Wednesdays and Saturdays. This type of routine requires a lot of time at the gym and is usually a workout reserved for the serious body builder. I don't believe this much time spent lifting weights will be required to reach your target weight loss goal.

Chest, Shoulder, and Triceps Workout (Mondays and Thursdays):

Bench Press - 4 sets of 8 repetitions

Flies - 4 sets of 8 repetitions

Dumbbell Military Press - 4 sets of 8 repetitions

Lateral Dumbbell Raises - 4 sets of 8 repetitions

Dips - 4 sets of 8 repetitions

Cable Triceps Press- 4 sets of 8 repetitions

Back and Bicep Workout (Tuesdays and Thursdays)

Wide Grip Lat Pull - 4 sets of 8 repetitions

Dumbbell Rows -4 sets of 8 repetitions

Barbell Rows - 4 sets of 8 repetitions

Barbell Curls - 4 sets of 8 repetitions

Standing Dumbbell Curls - 4 sets of 8 repetitions

Concentration Curls - 4 sets of 8 repetitions

Legs and Abs Workout (Wednesdays and Saturdays)

Squats - 4 sets of 8 repetitions

Calf Raises - 4 sets of 8 repetitions

Leg Press- 4 sets of 8 repetitions

Crunches - 4 sets of 25 repetitions

Leg Lifts - 4 sets of 8 repetitions

Leg Raises - 4 sets of 15 repetitions

Explanation of Exercises

Bench Press - is performed lying down on a weight bench. You place your hands approximately shoulder width apart. The movement is to lower the bar down until it touches your chest and then push it back up until your elbows are locked out.

Flies - are performed while lying on a bench and using dumbbells. Hold the dumbbells together above you with your elbows slightly bent. Spread the dumbbells apart in a lowering motion without changing the angle of your elbows. You should feel the burn in your pectoral muscles.

Military Press - is performed standing or sitting with either a barbell or with dumbbells. Start at the chest height position and press the weight above your head until the elbows lock out.

Lateral Dumbbell Raises - are performed with dumbbells in a standing position. Start with the weights hanging by your side and raise the weights till your arms are parallel with the floor without bending your elbows.

Dips - are performed on a set of dip bars. You suspend yourself with the elbows in the locked position. You then slowly lower your body by bending your elbows and then pushing yourself back up.

Cable Triceps Press- is done with a Lat machine. You stand upright and grab the bar around chin height. You then press the weight on the cable until your elbows are locked out.

Wide Grip Lat Pull - is performed with a Lat machine from a seated position and your legs braced to hold your body down. You grip the bar with a wider than shoulder width grip and pull the weight past your chin.

Barbell Rows - can be done with either a barbell or set of dumbbells. You bend at the waist with your knees slightly bent. Grab the weight and try to pull it to your chest.

Barbell Curls - are performed standing with a barbell or it can be performed with dumbbells as well. With your palms facing in front of you, grab the bar and curl it upward toward your chest.

Concentration Curls - are performed in a seated position with dumbbells. You will perform this exercise one arm at a time. Grab the dumbbell and let it hang in between your legs. Curl the dumbbell upward toward your chin.

Squats - are performed with a barbell behind your neck resting just below your traps and above the lats. From this position you will squat until hamstrings are parallel with the floor.

Calf Raises - can be done seated or standing with the weight either on top of your thighs or behind your neck. Raise your heels up and down to exercise the calf muscles.

Leg Press- is performed on a leg press machine. You will be in a seated position with your feet on the machine. You will press the weight in the same fashion as doing squats.

Crunches - is an ab exercise performed while lying down on your back with the knees slightly bent. With your hands behind your head, raise your head toward your toes thus exercising the ab muscles similar to a sit-up.

Leg Lifts - are performed on a bench with the leg lift attachment. From a seated position and your knees bent at a 90-degree angle you will lift the weight by straightening your legs.

Leg Raises - is an ab workout performed while lying flat on a bench. You grab a holt of the bench frame with your hands to stabilize and lift your feet in the air by bending at the waist.

Heavy Bag Training

Punching a heavy bag for me is a fun way to exercise. It can be a great way to relieve stress while getting an excellent upper body and cardio workout. All you will need is a heavy bag, a place to hang it securely, and some boxing gloves. I have really enjoyed my heavy bag workouts in the garage. You can download an app to your phone that will ring a bell to start and stop rounds. You can adjust the length of the rounds and the rest breaks. I like to perform ten rounds per workout. These rounds are set for one minute each with a 30 second break in between. Below is a sample workout

Round 1 - Left jabs

Round 2 - Right jabs

Round 3 - One then two combination (fighting righthanded)

Round 4 - One then two combination (fighting lefthanded or southpaw)

Round 5 - One, One then two combination

Round 6 - alternating uppercuts in the belly area

Round 7 - One, two, then Three combination

Round 8 - One then two combination with planned misses of the bag

Round 9 - One, two, then three combination with the three punch being a hook

Round 10 - Anything goes. Any combinations. Go all out for the final round

If you have the funds to purchase and a place to install a heavy bag you won't regret it. My heavy bag workouts have been so much fun. The workouts can really get your heart rate up for an excellent cardio session. It's also great self-defense training in case you were ever in a situation to where you had to defend yourself.

Chapter Five
Keeping Your Head in the Game

Results May Vary - Don't Get Discouraged

One thing I feel I need to point out is the speed you will get results. Don't get wrapped up in comparing yourself to my results or anyone else's. We all have a different rate in which we achieve results based mainly on our body type. One thing I learned from those old 1960's muscle magazines I used to read was on the three types of "Morphs" as I like to call them. This refers to the three-basic-types of body type in which we all as humans fit into. That's not to say that we all fit the template exactly but once you understand the basic concept you will find where you fit.

The first of these body types is the Ectomorph. The Ectomorph body type is one that is skinny or long and lean to be more exact. These folks typically have a high metabolism and find it difficult to make large gains in lean muscle. They typically make great track athletes and cross-country runners. I sometimes wish I could snap my fingers and become an ectomorph just before my 5K runs. I doubt there will be many of this body type purchasing my book because they typically don't have a weight issue and they can eat nearly anything in site without gaining a pound.

The next body type is the Mesomorph. This is the body type that I fit closer to. The Mesomorph is usually well built with the middle of the road metabolism. These are generally your athletes such as football players, wrestlers, body builders, etc. Mesomorphs can typically find it easier to gain lean muscle from working out with weights and other forms of training. That all sounds great, but the Mesomorph still needs to watch what they eat and keep their body moving or they will end up 50 lbs. overweight just as I was at the beginning of my journey.

The third and final body type is the Endomorph. The Endomorph is usually big with a high body fat percentage. You could compare their body shape to that of a pear. These folks typically have a slow metabolism and really have to watch what they eat and exercise regularly.

I hope I didn't hurt anyone's feelings with my interpretations of the three basic body types. That was not my intent. We are all created equal in the eyes of God, but we all have variations in our body type. I want you to have an understanding of this so that you won't compare yourself to someone of a different body type and expect the same results in the same time frame. I believe we can all achieve our goals if we work hard and stay focused.

Tracking Your Progress

There are many different ways to track your progress depending on the objective you plan to reach. Back in my strength training days the measure was maxing out periodically. We had max out days in weight training class usually about every month. We had three attempts at four different exercises to see how much weight we could lift. The four exercises or movements were Bench press, Squat, Deadlift and Power Clean. This is how our coach tracked our progress.

Runners, walkers and cyclists typically track their performance with distance and time. Body builders track overall size and proportion by taking measurements at different points on their body. Those of us inclined to lose weight can track our body fat percentage or simply step on a set of scales.

No matter what your objective, it is very important to keep track of your results on a weekly basis. This will help keep you motivated toward your goal. Weekly or even daily weigh ins help to ensure you're staying on track.

Depending on whatever your goal is, make sure you have your system of tracking progress set up on day one.

Following Through and Staying Focused

Following through and staying focused on your goal can be a challenge for all of us. The first time you miss a workout or give into the temptation of something not in your planned diet, it can be a stumbling block that brings you down. You may also experience a time during your journey in which you gain weight between weekly weigh-ins. This can be disheartening as well and can make you feel like giving up.

These things are only minimal, and they are probably going to happen over the course of your journey. All three of those things happened to me, but I didn't let it get me down. You have to stay focused on your goal when these hiccups happen. Whether it's losing weight or trying to gain muscle, it's mostly mental. Having the mental toughness to overcome obstacles will determine whether you succeed or fail in reaching your goal. I would venture to say that reaching a weight loss goal is 70 percent mental and 30 percent physical. There may be experts that disagree with that statement but I'm telling you to keep your head in the game and don't give up.

Napoleon Hill once said, "If you can conceive it and believe it, then you can achieve it." I believe that statement holds a lot of truth whether it's trying to lose weight or any other goal you can conceive.

Reaching Your Goal Weight and Maintaining a Healthy Lifestyle

The way I see it, there are two major parts to this fitness journey. The first part is reaching the goal weight that you set for yourself in the beginning. The second part is maintaining that goal weight and continuing a healthy lifestyle. Both of these parts require proper planning and execution to succeed.

In the past, losing weight for me has never been a problem. I'm good at getting motivated and putting a plan into action. These health kicks have usually failed because I didn't have a specific weight that I wanted to reach or a reason to maintain it once I got there. It's so easy to go back in the wrong direction if you don't plan accordingly.

I want you to have a specific reason that you desire to lose weight. It needs to be something bold and meaningful. The main reason I wanted to lose weight was so I could be healthier in years to come and prevent some of the health issues that could occur from being overweight. I also want to be around here on earth as long as I can to help raise and guide my children though their lives.

Reaching the goal weight that you set will be easier than maintaining it for the rest of your life. With that said, you will need to continue monitoring your weight and consuming a healthy diet. This means you will still need to step on the scales every few days and track where you are. Give yourself a five-pound window to work with. That's your "Red Flag mark". If you go over the Red Flag mark, then step up your cardio for a few days. It's all about managing your lifestyle and keeping things in check.

"I've failed over and over and over again in my life, and that is why I Succeed." -Michael Jordon

Chapter Six
My Final Journey

Overview of My Four-month Fitness Journey

As I have mentioned earlier, my journey started back during the Christmas holiday of 2018. One day in late December I stepped on the scales and found that I weighed over 285 lbs. That was the heaviest I had ever been in my life and it prompted me to make a change in my life. Being a man of 50 years old, I feared if I didn't make some drastic changes soon, I would be more susceptible to having health issues if I continued down the path I was on. Before the holidays were over, I had made up my mind and put together a detailed plan of attack for the new year. I've already explained in other chapters as to how I designed my plan and executed it. This chapter is for the purpose of showing you the results I tracked along the way and some of the foods I added to my diet.

<u>From sometime in mid-December to December 31st</u> I made up my mind to lose weight in the new year. During this time, I set my goal weight of 230 lbs. and designed a detailed plan of how I was going to achieve the goal.

<u>January 1st, 2019</u> - I weighed in at 286.6 lbs. On this day I made a video of my New Year's Resolution to lose weight and posted it on YouTube for everyone to see.

<u>January 2nd, 2019</u> - I walked for the first time. The length of the walk was just over one mile. I began executing my new diet with an emphasis on drinking water in place of all the soft drinks and sweet tea I had been consuming in the past.

<u>January 8th, 2019</u> - I weighed in at 271.8 lbs. This was a 14.8 lb. loss and largest one-week loss throughout my journey.

<u>January 15th, 2019</u> - I weighed in at 269.2 lbs.

<u>January 22nd, 2019</u> - I weighed in at 265.4 lbs.

<u>January 29th, 2019</u> - I weighed in at 262.2 lbs.

<u>January 31st, 2019</u> - End of the Month results. I weighed 259.8 lbs. which was an overall loss of 26.8 lbs. Over the course of the month I walked 60.8 miles. I also had several lightweight work outs and many 10 round sessions with the heavy bag.

<u>February 5th, 2019</u> - I weighed in at 257.4 lbs.

<u>February 12th, 2019</u> - I weighed in at 253.6 lbs.

<u>February 19th, 2019</u> - I weighed in at 249.6 lbs.

<u>February 26th, 2019</u> - I weighed in at 247.8 lbs.

<u>February 28th, 2019</u> - End of the Month results. I weighed in at 245.8 lbs. which was an overall loss of 40.8 lbs. Over the

course of this month I walked 82.3 miles. I didn't do a whole lot of weight training this month because I was mainly focusing on my walking. On some days I walked up to five miles at a time.

March 5th, 2019 - I weighed in at 243.8 lbs.

March 12th, 2019 - I weighed in at 241.4 lbs.

March 19th, 2019 - I weighed in at 239.0 lbs.

March 26th, 2019 - I weighed in at 239.2 lbs. Notice that I gained 0.2 lbs. during this week. You will have a week where that happens to you too so don't give up. Stay focused on the objective.

March 31st, 2019 - End of Month results. I weighed in at 235.2 lbs. which was an overall loss of 51.4 lbs. Over the course of this month I walked 60.1 miles and started incorporating some running into my workouts. By this date I had already signed up for a 5k run and was beginning to train for the event.

April 2nd, 2019 - I weighed in at 235.2 lbs.

April 9th, 2019 - I weighed in at 233.0 lbs.

April 13th, 2019 - I ran my first 5K event with an overall time of 35 minutes and 47 seconds. I finished 104th out of 152 people. No bad for my first attempt.

April 16th, 2019 - I weighed in at 231.8 lbs.

April 18th, 2019 - I REACHED MY GOAL WEIGHT OF 230.0 lbs. From this point on I set a five-pound window to maintain. 235 lbs. is the red flag mark that I want to stay under.

April 23rd, 2019 - I weighed in at 232.0 lbs.

<u>April 30th, 2019</u> - End of Month results. I weighed in at 229.6 lbs. which was an overall loss of 57 lbs. Over the course of this month I walked 47.7 miles. Since this date I have signed up for another 5K run in May and I'm currently working on this book so I can share it with the world and help others to a healthier lifestyle.

<u>May 7th, 2019</u> – I weighed in at 228.6 lbs.

I want to share with you what my diet consists of on a typical day. This may vary from day to day and I have on occasion enjoyed a burger from a local restaurant. I have learned to substitute a salad instead of French fries.

6:00am - A protein bar and 8oz. of Good ole Mountain Dew or Coke. This is only time during the day that I will drink a soft drink. The rest of the day I drink water.

8:00am to 9:00am - Workout (walking or running)

9:30am - Breakfast, a bowl of Granola or Raisin Bran cereal and some fruit (cantaloupe or watermelon)

12:00pm - A peanut butter and jelly sandwich. I usually have this on one slice of my homemade bread. Another choice I often have is two eggs scrambled with a slice of bacon.

3:00pm - A protein shake or a small serving of leftovers from the night before.

6:00pm - Dinner, typically a conservative portion of a meat, a starch such as rice or potatoes, and a green vegetable.

8:00pm - A protein shake or a protein bar.

Over the course of a day I probably drink a gallon or more of water and if I have any snacks in between meals its usually a piece of fruit (banana, apple, or an orange).

I want to also share with you a simple recipe for making homemade bread. I started making this bread for the health benefit of eliminating added preservatives and plus it tastes better than store bought bread.

My Homemade Bread Recipe

Ingredients:

3 slightly heaping Cups of all-purpose flour

1 and 1/2 Tablespoons of sugar

1 teaspoon of salt

1/4 of an ounce of fast acting Yeast

1 Cup of water

1/4 cup of milk

1 and 1/2 Tablespoons of butter or margarine

Add the water, milk, and butter into a small pot and place it on the stove at a low heat. This mixture needs to only reach 130 degrees. Typically, it's almost there when the butter melts.

Combine the rest of the ingredients into a large mixing bowl (flour, sugar, salt, and yeast). I like to use the tool for putting icing on a cake to mix the ingredients. When the liquids in the pot are at 130 degrees pour that mixture into the bowl of dry ingredients and start folding the mixture together. When the mixture is combined, and it doesn't stick to the tool anymore you can dump the dough into a well-greased 5" by 9" bread pan. Spread it out evenly, cover it, and let it rise for approximately 40 minutes. Don't let it go to long or it will start to fall. After is has risen I place it into a preheated oven at 400 degrees for 30 minutes. Take the bread out and let it cool completely before slicing. I have found that it slices best after cooling overnight. Another thing I like about this method of making bread is that you never have to get your hands in the dough. It goes straight from the mixing bowl to the pan. Clean-up is easy as well because very few kitchen tools are used in the process. I hope you enjoy making your own homemade bread as much as I do.

My First 5k Run

As I mentioned in a previous chapter, I began a strict regimen of walking daily back in January of this year. The results of walking daily had produced significant weight loss and a better feeling me. My leg strength and flexibility had improved tremendously.

It was on March 19th when I was driving to pick up my son from school that I noticed a banner on a street corner in town advertising a 5k Run. That sign got my attention and I thought about it the whole time I drove to pick up my son. On the way back, I pulled over and took a picture of the banner so I could google for more info when I got home.

After researching the event and finding out it was less than four weeks away, I decided to go for it. On March 20th, I registered online to make it official.

For those of you who don't know, a 5k run is equal to 3.1 miles. Even back in my football playing days I had never ran more than a mile or so at one time. I knew running a 5k would be a challenge but since I was already walking four to five miles on some days, I knew I could at least walk a 5k.

With less than four weeks to train, I began researching what others did to train for a 5k run. To my surprise I found a ton of info online and some really good videos on YouTube. The following day I started incorporating a slow jog into my daily walking route. I started in the neighborhood where I would jog the distance of two mailboxes and then walk to the next one. I repeated this over and over for the next several days. Then I began increasing the number of mailboxes until I could jog at least one lap around my neighborhood which is about a half of mile without stopping.

During this training process I did endure some difficulty in my 51-year-old body. My left knee and my right hip bothered me some, so I had to draw back the training in the days leading up to the race to let my body recover.

A few days before the race I began increasing my carb intake and drank a few bottles of Gatorade each day. On the morning of the race I had a protein bar when I first awoke. Then I had a slice of toast with peanut butter about an hour before race time.

My friend, Tina, rode with me to the event and filmed a nice video for my YouTube channel. After arriving and getting signed in we walked around and checked out the competition. There were folks from every age group and gender. I was amazed at the turnout on this dreary, chilly morning in April. I spent some time stretching and loosening up. I even had my picture taken with the Chick-fil-a Cow.

A few minutes before the start gun, I positioned myself near the rear of the field. I figured that most of these younger folks were faster than me and it would be best if I stayed out of their way. Soon we were off and running. To my surprise I made it almost to the first mile marker without having to stop and walk. By this time, the field had stretched out a bit and I was nowhere near the leaders, as expected, but I wasn't at the rear either. I kept trudging along alternating the walking with my jogging. Halfway through the third mile I got my second wind or rush of adrenalin in knowing that the race was concluding.

I went across the finish line with my friend Tina cheering me on. I finished my first 5k Run with a time of 35 minutes and 47 seconds. That was almost four minutes faster than my best practice run leading up to the days event.

After the race we stayed and watched the awards ceremony as I envied the winners in each class. Needless to say, I didn't bring home any metals on that day, but my reward was the fact that I had completed a 5k Run and did it without injury.

All in all, this was a great experience and I'm already planning on running another 5k later this year. I highly recommend that everyone should enter at least one 5k Run, even if you can only walk it. It's a great experience and most of these events sponsor a good charitable cause.

"If something stands between you and success. Move it. Never

be Denied." -Dwayne "The Rock" Johnson

Chapter Seven
The Game Plan & Final Thoughts

Game Plan

Have you ever read a "how to" book and at the end you wondered "where do I start?" Most books give you pages and pages of information, but they never give you an exact plan to execute whatever the subject may be. Well, I am going to change all of that in this chapter. I'm going to give you a detailed Game Plan to follow. Unlike a head football coach that keeps his game plan on a clipboard and paces the sidelines, I will reveal a template below that you can use to create your own personal Game Plan for your fitness journey.

1) Consult a physician to evaluate this information and help determine if this program is right for you.

2) Make Time for You- Find at least a one-hour time slot that is for just you every day.

3) Set a Specific Goal Weight that you want to reach.

4) Plan your Diet- Don't eliminate any foods or drinks that you enjoy but plan on their reduction and frequency in your new meal plan. Add healthier options to your diet, such as fruits and vegetables. Split your meals into several smaller meals and practice portion control at every meal. Don't Go Hungry!

5) Exercise- Figure out what type of exercises you are going to execute in your journey. Have all necessary equipment and clothing planned out before your start date. You will perform whatever exercise you choose during your daily personal time block.

6) Official Weigh In- On your first weigh-in, I want you to do it in the evening after you have consumed most of your daily food and liquids. You can also be fully dressed for this weigh-in as well. I want this weigh-in to look BAD, because this is your starting point in which all progress will be measured. After this weigh-in you will track an official weigh-in every seven days. These remaining weigh-ins will be performed in the morning wearing nothing but your underwear. You will experience the biggest weight loss in the first week of this program. I want it to be impressive so it will help motivate you to continue and work even harder.

7) Tell Everyone- I want you to announce to everyone you know that you are going to lose weight and change your

lifestyle. Tell your close friends, family, and post it all over social media so you can be held accountable. This will also help to motivate you to continue and succeed.

8) Remember that Losing Weight and Changing your lifestyle is mostly mental. Your body will follow along with whatever you tell it to do. It's your mindset that needs to change. Stay focused on the objective.

9) Get Tough and Don't Make Excuses- Your body is tougher that you give it credit for. You will experience some muscle soreness in the beginning so don't make that a reason to quit and give up. It will pass just as my shin splints did back in high school from the two-a-day football practices I endured. Don't make excuses for not exercising! Remember the story I told you about the 80-year-old lady walking on a 23-degree day. You have no excuse!

10) Reach the Goal you Set- It is important that you reach your target goal weight. This will mark the completion of a major accomplishment. Don't fall five-pounds short and say that's good enough. I want you to reach the goal that you projected.

11) Execute your New Lifestyle- Now that you have reached your goal you don't get a free pass to stop exercising and go back to sitting on the sofa eating Bon Bons. I want you to analyze your diet and exercise over the past weeks and make adjustments to where you can continue to maintain the weight that you have lost. This could mean that you can increase your calorie intake some or cut back on the cardio. Give yourself a

five-pound window to manage and make adjustments in your diet and exercise to maintain this weight.

12) Now put this plan to use and Go Make It Happen!

Ready, Set Go

Folks, I've given you everything I know about the subject of weight loss and fitness in this book. This is not some easy, microwave fast, instant weight loss program. This is just common sense, good old-fashioned hard work and perseverance. You can do this if you believe in yourself. If you truly want to change your body and your overall health this is the way.

Make this the final time in your life that you have to lose weight. Donate all your fat clothes to Goodwill and welcome in the new lifestyle change that awaits you.

Now Get Ready!

Set!

and GO FOR IT!!!!!!!